Mind Diet

Enhance Your Desires, Enhance Cognitive Function
And Indulge In A More Blissful Existence With Nutritional
Dishes From The Mind Diet

*(The Definitive 21-day Dietary Program For Enhancing
Cognitive Function In The Battle Against Alzheimer's
Disease And Dementia)*

Alfred Dietrich

TABLE OF CONTENT

Introduction.. 1
   What Is the MIND Diet?................................... 1
It Is Highly Probable That You Are Familiar With The Renowned Quotation Attributed To Hippocrates. 18
Hamburgers And French Fries Are Available. ... 53
You're Body 76
An Understanding Of The End Date 98
Greek Yogurt Breakfast Bowl 123
A Selection Of Food Items To Incorporate Into The Mind Diet.. 124

Introduction

WHAT IS THE MIND DIET?

The combination of the DASH and Mediterranean diets has been thoroughly evaluated by experts, who regard it as a robust and formidable dietary regimen. Research studies have demonstrated that these dietary patterns have exhibited a beneficial effect on various chronic illnesses, encompassing the reduction of blood pressure, mitigated risk of cardiovascular conditions, and diminished susceptibility to diabetes, among others.

To explicitly aim at enhancing cognitive abilities and mitigating the risk of dementia, scientists have devised a diet with this precise objective in mind. In order to achieve this, they amalgamated principles from the Mediterranean and DASH dietary patterns that have been demonstrated to enhance cognitive capacity.

This integrated nutritional regimen advocates for the consumption of berries due to a proven cause-and-effect relationship linked to enhanced cognitive capacities. The dietary guidelines for individuals also advocate for a substantial consumption of fruits, despite the absence of any established correlation with enhanced cognitive well-being. The MIND diet promotes the consumption of berries while not placing significant emphasis on the consumption of fruits in general.

No formal protocol for adhering to the MIND diet has been established. Nevertheless, the diet advocates for the consumption of specific food items while discouraging the incorporation of Five (5) into one's daily routine.

Ranking the 10 most effective foods for enhancing cognitive function

The MIND diet advocates for the consumption of the following 10 foods:

Beans:

This particular food item ought to be incorporated into a minimum of four meals per week. This dietary plan advocates for the inclusion of all legumes, including beans, peas, lentils, and soybeans.

Berries:

It is recommended to incorporate this food into a minimum of two meals on a weekly basis. Although the published research exclusively pertains to strawberries, it is advisable to consider incorporating other berries such as blueberries, raspberries, and blackberries into the discussion of their antioxidant benefits.

Fish:

Consuming this food on a weekly basis is recommended. Consider incorporating fish varieties such as sardines, salmon, mackerel, trout, or tuna into your diet, as they boast significant levels of omega-3 fatty acids.

Green leafy vegetables:

Strive to incorporate a minimum of 6 portions of green leafy vegetables into your weekly diet. This encompasses an assortment of leafy greens such as kale, spinach, and various varieties of cooked greens. In addition to these vegetables, it is essential to incorporate other varieties of vegetables into our daily consumption. Non-starchy vegetables are highly appropriate due to their abundant nutritional content and significantly reduced caloric value.

Nuts:

Try to consume a minimum of 5 servings of nuts per week. A diverse assortment of nuts ought to be incorporated.

Olive oil:

This food is recommended for utilization as your primary cooking oil.

Poultry:

This food ought to be incorporated into one's diet at a minimum of twice per week. Consumption of fried chicken is not advised within the parameters of this diet.

Whole grains:

It is recommended to consume this food in a minimum of three servings per day. Incorporate entire grains such as quinoa, oatmeal, brown rice, 100% whole-wheat bread, and whole-wheat pasta.

Wine:

The consumption of both red and white wine can have a positive impact on brain health. Nevertheless, the primary area of interest for the majority of researchers lies in examining the resveratrol compound present in red wine, as it possesses the ability to combat the development of Alzheimer's disease. It is advisable to limit the consumption of one glass per day.

Other Veggies

The MIND diet, as well as any well-rounded diet, places importance on the consumption of vegetables, particularly leafy greens, at approximately one serving per day. Additionally, the MIND diet advocates for incorporating a variety of vegetable types on a daily basis. It need not be arduous. Incorporate tomatoes and red pepper strips into sandwiches and sauté them alongside broccoli and cauliflower. Enhance pasta dishes with nutritious vegetable noodles such as zucchini or carrot noodles. Alternatively, enjoy them as a snack with cherry tomatoes and hummus.

The following are the dietary restrictions imposed by the MIND diet:

1. Red Meat

Red meat exhibits a higher fat content in comparison to alternative protein sources, such as poultry or tofu. Additionally, a separate investigation amalgamated a rise in cerebral iron levels with an elevated susceptibility to Alzheimer's disease, indicating that the consumption of copious amounts of red meat may potentially contribute as a causative agent.

2. Deep-fried and Rapid-Service Cuisine

Numerous deep-fried food items contain excessive levels of unhealthy saturated fats, much like various other fast food options.

3. Whole-Fat Cheese

Consume no more than one portion per week. The cheese contains a significant amount of saturated fat. Although you may have acquired the knowledge that processed cheese containing aluminum metal could potentially elevate the likelihood of developing dementia, recent research has negated the notion that minuscule amounts of aluminum derived from food contribute to an increased risk of Alzheimer's disease.

4. Butter /Margarine

A maximum limit of one tablespoon per day should not be exceeded. Butter is rich in saturated fats, whereas vegetable oil, such as soybean oil used for omega-6 fats, comprises margarine. An excessive intake of omega-6 fatty acids has the potential to promote heightened levels of inflammation.

5. Pastries and Sweets

A limit of up to five servings per week. In addition, these treats contain significant amounts of both saturated fat and sugar. Additionally, sugar has the ability to stimulate the reward system within the body, thereby triggering a heightened desire for increased consumption.

Breakfast Recipes

If one is committed to adhering to a nutritious dietary plan, it is imperative to make judicious selections when it comes to food consumption. The culinary offerings at this establishment have been specially crafted to cater to your breakfast requirements. Each culinary formula possesses distinctive components that confer nutritional advantages. Consequently, commencing your day with these meals guarantees a nourishing and invigorating experience. Please peruse them and relish the experience.

Resolve to change. Do not dwell on matters of dietary restriction and

exercise

Initially, the most challenging aspect of shedding the excess weight

The act of arriving at this particular choice may be within your purview.

Conceived a weight loss plan beforehand, yet failed to execute it.

Fail, potentially due to your lack of unwavering determination.

Initially, it is imperative to ascertain your willingness to voluntarily relinquish a portion of

What specific provisions are you currently seeking, such as pre-prepared meals, in order to optimize the situation?

in subsequent times (a state of well-being and balanced physical condition) and thereafter

If you steadfastly adhere to this intention, the outcome will be the attainment of weight loss.

an easy process.

2

Weigh yourself. If your current weight is unknown, it is advisable to weigh yourself at your residence using a balance or at a conveniently located pharmacy. It is crucial to possess knowledge of your initial weight while embarking upon your endeavor to shed excess weight, as this will enable you to effectively monitor your progress.

progress.

Utilize a digital weighing scale to obtain precise measurements.

The optimal moment to measure your weight is in the early morning prior to your first meal.

Consume any kind of nourishment while adorned in lightweight attire.

For the purpose of effective muscle building, it can be advantageous to occasionally measure the circumferences of specific body parts such as the arm, leg, chest, waist, and buttocks, or any area targeted for weight loss. This will enable you to monitor the centimeters lost, while considering the potential muscle mass that could replace the lost weight, as muscles tend to be denser than fat.

3

Decrease the caloric intake. When it comes to

Weight loss largely hinges upon adhering to the dietary regimen, which represents a paramount aspect.

You are required to attend to, as the caloric intake decreases, the...

The more weight you shed, it is as straightforward as that. It is also important

to ensure adequate nourishment and supply you with the necessary sustenance

Fundamental dietary components, and refrain from contemplating deprivation.

By refraining from indulging in this behavior, you can actively mitigate the intensification of your desires and prevent a relapse.

Ultimately, the negative dietary practices you possess.

Numerous medical professionals maintain the perspective that consuming a daily intake of 1200 calories

on a daily basis, irrespective of your present weight, will result in a

Progressive reduction in your body mass. It is likely to require a certain amount of time to

Understand the recommended caloric intake for your daily needs

Relative to the weight reduction observed on the weighing scale.

Persist with an iterative process while fine-tuning the quantity of

Consume the food until you achieve the optimal caloric intake suitable for your individual body composition.

Commence the practice of meticulously monitoring the caloric content of all food items consumed, even in inconspicuous quantities.

food items that are typically disregarded and not given due attention

Take into account noteworthy items, such as dressings for salads, carbonated beverages, and

cooking oil. Please peruse the nutritional details provided on the packaging or label of the food item.

purchased bundles, and compute your daily

The stipulation that applies to all of them on a daily basis. You can use the

"The internet platforms exemplified by Calorie King and My Fitness Pal" to

Conduct a comprehensive analysis of the calorie content in fruits, vegetables, and meat

does not possess a label indicating its nutritional content.

4

Engage in physical activity on a regular basis, approximately 4-5 times per week. Aerobic exercises that

Elevating the heart rate can lead to the burning of calories and augmentation.

The metabolic rate experiences a temporary increase within a few hours following each instance.

Physical activity, hence the physical exercises expedite the

process of losing weight. [1] Remember that exercise

Solely relying on one's own efforts would not lead to weight loss. [2] It is imperative for you to alter your

Modifying dietary practices is imperative for weight loss.

Physical activities of an aerobic nature, such as engaging in a running exercise regimen,

walking, swimming

Furthermore, engaging in activities such as walking, running, and cycling prove to be highly effective exercises for calorie expenditure and

Enhance overall well-being, particularly if you are unaccustomed to it.

When initiating a fitness routine, it is imperative to begin gradually until mastery is achieved.

Engaging in the practice, and it is imperative that you discover a

The sport that you are particularly fond of, in order to facilitate physical activity.

daily.

It Is Highly Probable That You Are Familiar With The Renowned Quotation Attributed To Hippocrates.

I strongly adhere to the notion that nutrition serves as both a remedy and nourishment, as echoed by the famous adage, "Let food be thy medicine and medicine be thy food." Food acts as a source of sustenance for our physical well-being, furnishing us with both vital energy and essential nutrients that can either contribute to the maintenance of our health or impede it. Additionally, it fulfills the role of a caretaker by addressing our emotional well-being, encompassing our cultural heritage, and connecting with our individual life experiences. In my capacity as a professional dietitian and culinary expert, I am deeply committed to integrating the nutritional and nurturing elements of food through the art of cooking.

In matters concerning nutrition, one tends to consume healthier foods when they personally engage in their preparation. Engaging in culinary activities allows individuals to exercise meticulous oversight over the nutritional content they consume, thereby imparting a heightened level of authority in tailoring their dietary regimen to align with their personal health requisites and aspirations. When it concerns matters of health, both in terms of prevention and management of conditions, adhering to a therapeutic diet and practicing proper nourishment can have a profound impact. Acquiring the skill of preparing nutritious meals at home is an excellent strategy to cultivate a foundation for achieving positive outcomes.

Cooking can provide emotional therapy as well; it can be gratifying to create a meal for your loved ones as a means of demonstrating your care for them. There is no feeling quite as gratifying as experiencing a profound sense of pride derived from crafting a delectable dish using uncomplicated, wholesome ingredients that exude delightful aromas and tantalize the taste buds. You establish a more profound rapport with the food you consume when you engage in its personal preparation. The establishment of such a profound bond can contribute to the enhancement of your relationship with food.

I have been fortunate to witness the convergence of the nutritional and nurturing dimensions of cooking. Over the course of multiple years, I held the position of leading a teaching kitchen initiative at an esteemed academic medical center. During my tenure, I successfully conceptualized and implemented a range of programs aimed at instructing patients on the nuances of preparing meals to adhere to their prescribed therapeutic diets. This encompassed the implementation of ketogenic culinary practices for individuals suffering from epilepsy, the adoption of low-FODMAP and gluten-free culinary approaches for patients with digestive health issues, and the integration of low-protein cooking techniques for individuals afflicted with phenylketonuria, more commonly referred to as PKU—a severe genetic disorder that impedes the metabolism of specific amino acids. Additionally, I have designed and instructed culinary education programs targeted at promoting cardiovascular well-being, controlling diabetes, achieving weight reduction objectives, enhancing overall health through better nutrition practices, and providing comprehensive culinary advice. I observed a significant transformation among individuals who initially felt apprehensive about culinary endeavors, even expressing reluctance towards the notion of preparing daily meals for their families. However, they gradually acquired confidence in using knives, adopting basic cooking techniques, and organizing meals, thus reflecting a notable growth in their culinary skills. As a practitioner in the field of nutrition and food, few things bring me greater gratification than witnessing individuals prioritize their well-being by engaging in culinary practices, and observing the subsequent positive alterations in their physical well-being and overall life quality.

Alzheimer's is an incapacitating and calamitous illness. Diligent efforts have been made by investigators to discover remedies and therapies, and scholarly inquiry suggests that sustenance and life practices assume a fundamental role in inhibiting cognitive decline. I have come here with the intention of assisting you in implementing the research findings and suggestions pertaining to the MIND diet. This diet, known for its efficacy in lowering the likelihood of developing

Alzheimer's disease and dementia, will be translated into practical applications within your culinary endeavors. In a similar manner as I did with my patients within the instructional culinary setting, I aim to demonstrate to you the techniques and practices of cooking and consuming meals that lower the probability of developing Alzheimer's disease and dementia. I trust that this book will not only serve as a source of inspiration, but will also elucidate the profound influence of food on the overall well-being of your mind and body.

Implementing the MIND Diet in Practice

According to Vandana R., "The MIND diet is a relatively straightforward diet to adhere to." Ms.Sheth, a Registered Dietitian Nutritionist (RDN) and Certified Diabetes Educator (CDE), serves as a representative for the prestigious Academy of Nutrition and Dietetics. It abstains from providing explicit nutrient recommendations in favor of broader dietary patterns. According to Sheth, maintaining a daily consumption of a green salad and another variety of vegetables, along with incorporating nuts as a snack, is a relatively effortless endeavor. A significant portion of the population already consumes poultry at least twice a week in addition to partaking in a glass of wine during dinner or prior to retiring for the evening. Incorporating fish on a weekly basis can be as effortless as including a can of tuna in one's lunch salad.

Consuming three portions of whole grains on a daily basis might appear challenging; nevertheless, it is essential to remind patients that just a single slice of bread can be considered a serving. Hence, this objective can be achieved by opting for oatmeal during breakfast and a sandwich made with whole grain bread for lunch, or by consuming a bowl of whole grain cereal in the morning and a cup of brown rice or barley soup for dinner. Berries can be quite costly, especially when not in season, but frozen berries offer the same nutritional value as fresh berries and are excellent when added to oatmeal or used in smoothies and yogurt parfaits throughout the entire year. Beans present an ideal option for individuals who eschew cooking, adhere to a strict financial plan, or encounter challenges with dental conditions. Canned beans that have been rinsed can be added to salads, incorporated into prepared soups, stews, and chilies, or served over brown rice with some basic herbs and spices for a nutritionally beneficial meal.

Reducing the consumption of saturated fats poses a significant challenge for many Americans. Transitioning gradually from whole milk to 2%, and subsequently to 1% over a period of time, proves to be an effective approach. It may pose a challenge to abstain from consuming cheese, to restrict the intake of red and processed meats, and to adhere to a maximum of one tablespoon of butter per day. Similarly, reducing the consumption of pastries, cookies, and other sugary treats may prove to be a formidable task for numerous individuals. It might be beneficial to consider dessert as an exceptional indulgence rather than a necessity for completing a meal. "It is imperative to acknowledge that modifying behavior poses a challenging task," states Sheth. A diet should not be viewed as a temporary plan; instead, it should be seen as a lasting alteration to one's lifestyle. Effective strategies often involve focusing on a few manageable objectives at a time. By incorporating healthy options such as salads, whole grains, fish, and beans, individuals can displace some of the less advisable choices from their diet. Assure patients that any progression towards the optimal dietary pattern is a beneficial measure for both neurological and cardiovascular well-being. According to Morris, one of the advantages of the MIND diet is that individuals can still experience benefits even if they do not strictly adhere to its guidelines.

According to Sheth, elderly individuals frequently encounter additional factors that further complicate the process of making sound dietary decisions. \"Proper nutrition allows us to prevent, delay, and effectively manage both the natural aging process and chronic conditions,\" she states. \"However, elderly individuals frequently encounter physical, emotional, and social transformations that impact their capacity to maintain a healthy diet.\ These factors encompass limited capacity to shop, prepare, and cook meals; financial constraints; a lack of motivation to cook; changes in taste and appetite due to medications and normal aging; and difficulties with chewing or swallowing. Healthcare professionals who work with this population are well-positioned to assess these issues while delivering other necessary care. According to Sheth, engaging in a conversation about dietary habits and the significance of adequate nutrition, while also considering the possibility of referring to a registered dietitian if needed, can yield significant positive outcomes.

As the field of nutrition and cognitive neuroscience continues to develop, a wealth of increasingly precise data is anticipated to emerge. It is evident, even at this stage, that lifestyle modifications concerning diet can confer neuroprotective effects and should be promoted in individuals. According to Sheth, the incorporation of the MIND diet principles can have a beneficial impact not only on the neurological health of elderly patients, but also on their overall well-being and general health.

RUNNING

Running represents the initial physical activity performed by humans. How? In the pursuit of securing sustenance, humankind would engage in the activity of hunting, which necessitated a physical effort to pursue and capture animals. Engaging in a 30-minute running session yields a higher caloric expenditure compared to engaging in a weight training regimen of equal duration at the gym.

Just as cheese serves as the primary component in the recipe for pizza, running functions as the central element within our program. Does the mention of pizza currently ignite a sense of temptation within you? I know. It occurred to me while I was in the process of writing. Regardless, let us redirect our attention to the subject at hand. Therefore, as stipulated in the 30-Day Guided Weight Loss Program, it is mandatory to engage in a daily running routine.

Engaging in solitary running yields a multitude of advantages that surpass those offered by alternative forms of physical activity. Research indicates that individuals who engage in running tend to have a longer lifespan in comparison to those who do not participate in this activity. Engaging in vigorous physical exercise enhances cardiovascular health and fortifies the skeletal system. It boosts your mood. There exist numerous rationales for commencing a consistent running practice and incorporating it into your daily routine. Let us shift our attention towards the specific kind of jogging required for this program.

One must engage in running on the roadway or pathway amidst the expanse of the uncovered atmosphere. Refrain from engaging in physical activity on the treadmill. The duration of running and the distance covered will incrementally escalate on a daily basis.

Engaging in a morning jog is the most optimal approach to running. If one resides within the urban vicinity, the presence of pollution will be diminished and there will be a reduced number of vehicles traversing the roadways. Residing in rural areas grants individuals the opportunity to inhale unpolluted air during the early hours of the day. Insufficient intake of vitamin D is often observed. However, engaging in morning runs will also yield advantageous outcomes for your skeletal system.

We shall adhere to a daily regimen, incorporating two intervals for physical exercise.

Embark on a journey (D)-Relocating from one's residence without notifying authorities or guardians

Arrival - Hastening towards Residency

Let's assume that your objective for today's run is to cover a distance of 4 miles. Next, you will be required to commence your run from your residence towards your intended endpoint, covering a distance of 2 miles. This shall be regarded as your Departure (D) distance. Following this, you will then be expected to return to your home, covering a further 2 miles, which will be classified as your Arrival (A) distance.

How should I run?

Stretching:

It is imperative to engage in a daily routine of stretching before engaging in a running session. One may engage in a comprehensive, whole-body stretching routine lasting approximately 4 to 5 minutes. It can aid in the alleviation of muscle tension, enabling a smooth running experience devoid of any discomfort or rigidity.

A limited number of my clients expressed a preference for walking as opposed to running. Their prevalent query constituted, 'Is it permissible to engage in brisk walking as an alternative to running?' To which the response provided was in the negative.

Regardless of your walking speed, this program requires you to run. You are permitted to maintain a leisurely pace while running, but it is mandatory that you engage in running. Engaging in any form of walking does not yield any benefits within the context of this program.

As you advance in this program, your running distance will gradually augment. Suppose your objective for running is to cover a distance of 3 miles. In the event that you experience fatigue following a 1.5-mile run, it is recommended to engage in a leisurely walk spanning a distance ranging from 300 to 500 meters, allowing for a period of rest and recuperation. After replenishing your energy, you may resume your running activity.

The focus of this program lies on the distance covered rather than the velocity of your running. The attainment of your running goal is of utmost importance. The pace of running, whether it is slow, moderate, or fast, is inconsequential. I defer to your judgment regarding the speed. You have the freedom to run at a pace that is personally comfortable to you. Furthermore, it is advisable to engage in periods of relaxation when you experience fatigue. In addition, you can achieve relaxation through engaging in a short stroll. Regardless of the nature of the task, it is imperative that you traverse the distance. This ought to be your primary goal.

One can utilize a fitness smartwatch or install a fitness application on a smartphone to accurately monitor the distance covered during a running session. Please be reminded that these tools are intended solely for the purpose of measuring distances, and there is no need to delve into the intricacies of caloric expenditure. Additionally, a waist pouch or small backpack may be employed for the purpose of running. This pouch has the capacity to accommodate various items like a water bottle, skipping rope, mobile phone, and so on. However, it is important to note that during physical activity, such as running, it is crucial that the waist pouch, backpack, and their contents remain stationary and do not experience any sort of bouncing or jumping. It is essential that the item is securely fastened to your body, thereby ensuring a seamless running experience without encountering any difficulties.

Our initial activity will be to cover a distance of 0.5 miles on the inaugural day, after which we will systematically augment the distance in accordance with our advancements. On the thirtieth day, you will engage in a running session covering a distance of 10 miles. Despite the gradual increment in distance over a span of 30 days, the physical act of running poses a formidable challenge, particularly for individuals who lack prior experience or inclination towards it as a form of exercise. In order to achieve that, it will be necessary to possess a considerable degree of determination, commitment, and willingness to make personal sacrifices.

The 10 Miles Marathon serves as the optimal method to sustain motivation over the course of 30 days. Numerous marathons are being organized within your urban vicinity. One may opt to participate in any 10-mile marathon event of their choice approximately one month from now and make an advance registration for the same. Should your city not be chosen as a host for a marathon, rest assured that there exist numerous options for participating in virtual marathons. This objective can be achieved by undertaking a 10-mile run within your local municipality or rural area on that designated day, subsequent to which you would be required to provide visual proof, such as a photograph or screenshot, attesting to the completion of the race within the specified timeframe. Subsequently, the medal will be dispatched to you via courier. That shall serve as your recompense.

Your guiding principle is to diligently ready oneself in anticipation of that forthcoming occasion, scheduled to occur within a month. It is imperative that you actively participate in the 10-mile race alongside your fellow participants and complete it with a sense of accomplishment. The objective of equipping oneself for a 10-mile marathon will serve as a continual source of motivation during the entirety of this 30-Day Guided Weight Loss Program.

3/

MY METHOD

I will be presenting techniques that others typically charge exorbitant sums of money to access. I shall elucidate the precise methodology through which I have assisted numerous individuals in attaining the pinnacle of their physical well-being. Instead of delving into the nuanced intricacies of the programs, I shall prioritize elucidating the significant impact of your mental faculties on your fitness objectives.

The predominant factor contributing to obesity in contemporary society is the phenomenon of 'unconscious eating'. The singular fact, which serves as the foremost lesson I have acquired in my capacity as a fitness professional, is as follows: should we consume food absentmindedly, the outcome shall invariably be

Cultivate an unhealthy dietary habit

I tend to consume excessive quantities of food, and

I have gained excess weight as a consequence of this.

This phenomenon is commonly referred to as "mindless eating." I have discovered that the greater the cognitive clarity one possesses, the more conscientious one becomes. The greater level of consciousness you possess, the more effectively you will adhere to a substantial fitness regimen.

As you are likely aware, I have faced the ongoing challenge of dealing with excess weight for an extended period of time, during which I made various attempts to address it through multiple diet and exercise regimens, all of which proved ineffective. No other solution proved as effective for me as the knowledge I am about to impart to you.

One notable revelation that I encountered was the observation that each of us consistently engages in erratic thinking. Our thoughts are scattered and unfocused. We frequently contemplate the past and consistently harbor concerns regarding the future. On average, our cognitive processes generate around 60,000 thoughts per day, with a significant portion of these thoughts being rendered superfluous and characterized by repetition. Indeed, a significant proportion of them exhibit negative characteristics.

It is disconcerting to acknowledge that our thoughts can contribute to weight gain. Acclaimed science writer Gary Taubes highlights this concept in his best-selling diet book, "Why We Get Fat," which expounds upon the notion that the mere contemplation of carbohydrates can elevate insulin levels and lead to the accumulation of excess fat. Our society is experiencing an increase in obesity not solely due to dietary habits, but rather as a result of cognitive factors.

Furthermore, these contemplations obfuscate our authentic identities as, in actuality, the present point in time encompasses our sole existence. At this present moment, while you engage in the act of perusing the words imprinted upon this page, it is, in fact, the entirety of our currently available information. This moment!

An immense quantity of information vies for our attention, totaling in the billions of bits. Regrettably, on numerous occasions, our attention is not directed towards the appropriate matters. However, these cognitions, sentiments, and affective states do contribute to our tendency to consume excessive amounts of food.

Furthermore, we engage in rationalization regarding our lack of exercise. We are currently experiencing a significant level of activity. Each individual is occupied.

Upon inquiring with my clients as to the reason for their infrequent exercise routine, the common response I receive is that they are unable to dedicate sufficient time due to their busy schedules.

May I inquire as to why you are not consuming nutritious food?

Their response is, "due to the significant time required for preparation, I am unable to allocate the necessary time."

These beliefs are simply restrictive in nature. As we progress together, I am committed to dispelling any inhibitive convictions that hinder your pursuit of optimal health and fitness.

According to John Maxwell, an individual can sustain their life for a span of 40 days sans sustenance, 4 days without hydration, and a mere 4 minutes without the vital resource of air. However, it is asserted that the indispensable element of Hope can only be withdrawn for a fleeting 4 seconds before its profound absence becomes acutely felt.

Nick Sisman was employed as a member of a railway crew. Nick appeared to possess all the trappings that one might desire: a spousal partner, two robust offspring, a respectable occupation, and a wide network of acquaintances.

Nevertheless, Nick possessed a single flaw. He had gained a reputation for being an infamous worrier. He was plagued by constant concerns and typically harbored apprehensions of dire outcomes.

On a particular summer day, the train crew received notification that they had the option to conclude their duties one hour earlier as a gesture to commemorate the foreman's birthday. Inadvertently, after the remaining workers departed the location, Nick found himself confined within a refrigerated boxcar.

Nervousness overcame Nick as he frantically pounded and vociferously called out, resulting in severely bruised knuckles and a strained vocal cords. No one heard him.

He pondered upon the chilling fate that awaited him if he failed to find an escape route. In an earnest effort to communicate the events that had befallen him to his wife and family, Nick procured a knife and proceeded to meticulously inscribe words onto the surface of the wooden flooring.

He wrote:

The extremely low temperature is causing a loss of sensation in my body. If I could simply retire for the night, this message might perhaps be my final utterance...

On the subsequent morning, as the crew cautiously slid apart the weighty doors of the boxcar, they discovered the lifeless body of Nick. Upon examination, it was determined through an autopsy that the deceased had succumbed to hypothermia, as evidenced by the various physical indicators on his body. It is perplexing, however, to note that despite the malfunctioning refrigeration unit in the car, the internal temperature remained consistently mild at fifty-five degrees.

Crazy, right?

This narrative imparts the profound lesson that the human intellect possesses remarkable strength and influence.

The human mind possesses such extraordinary potency that it has the ability to persuade an individual of ideas that lack veracity.

I have come across a research paper elucidating the relationship between cognitive processes and the physiological mechanisms governing weight gain and loss. The thesis examines the correlation between a designated cognitive framework and its potential impact on one's body weight, suggesting that said pattern of thinking may be associated with a tendency towards being slimmer. The aforementioned statement implies that you are possibly engaging in thoughts that have the potential to result in weight gain.

Alternatively, maintaining an awareness of the fact that you are engaging in physical activity can result in enhanced fitness levels.

In the month of February, in the year 2007, a scientific investigation conducted by Harvard University and published in the journal Psychological Science monitored the well-being of a cohort consisting of 84 female room attendants employed across multiple hotels. The study unveiled that women who acknowledged their physical activity as "exercise" realized noteworthy improvements in their overall health.

The females were divided into two distinct groups.

A specific cohort was informed that their daily work effectively met all the prescribed daily activity levels for maintaining good health. The remaining group of women, referred to as the "control group," proceeded with their tasks in their typical manner without being privy to this information.

Despite the fact that neither group altered their behavior, the women who were mindful of their activity level witnessed a substantial reduction in weight, blood pressure, body fat, waist-to-hip ratio, and body mass index within a mere four-week period.

The group designated as the "control group" did not exhibit any health enhancements, despite their participation in identical physical activities.

This research showcases the significant impact that one's attitude can have on their physical health.

It is truly astonishing how mere awareness of one's participation in a transformation program and making a minor adjustment in one's mindset can produce profound outcomes!

Renowned psychologist Abraham Maslow, recognized globally for his expertise, formulated his own hierarchical model of needs. In this conceptual framework, he discerned the fundamental requirements common to all individuals. Without the fulfillment of a particular primary requirement, an individual will never be able to proceed to their subsequent necessity. The theory is characterized by its simplicity and is thoroughly elucidated in Maslow's seminal research, wherein he intricately examines these individual needs:

► Food

► Shelter

► Love

► Lastly, the topic of family emerges.

► Self-Actualization

Likewise, your endeavors towards achieving optimal health and fitness will remain unattainable unless you have adequately addressed these fundamental requisites.

This is the juncture where the psychological components of weight management and physical well-being come into operation. Provided that your mental state is stable and all aspects of your well-being are coordinated, you will be incapable of directing your attention towards your physical fitness and health in the same astute manner that would be achievable once those essential necessities are satisfactorily fulfilled.

Therefore, please ensure that you bear that in mind. First and foremost, it is imperative to attend to the inner game by ensuring that one is fully focused and attuned to oneself. Subsequently, and solely after achieving a state of inner harmony and self-acceptance, you can employ the potent concepts of mindful consumption.

That statement holds great depth of meaning.

I will present a multitude of influential tactical insights that will aid you in attaining optimal physical well-being. I will impart numerous similar insights to you, and offer you a practical demonstration of their application towards accomplishing your fitness objectives.

Our physical beings are composed of three fundamental constituents:

▶ what we eat,

▶ the beverages we consume, and

▶ what we think.

Cognitive processes, or our mental faculties, play a pivotal role in our physical well-being.

Reflect upon this inquiry: what is the reason behind the absence of overweight creatures in the natural world? The sole creatures exhibiting obesity are exclusively those that have been domesticated or are held captive within a zoo environment. Put simply, the obese animals refer to those that primarily dwell in close proximity to humans.

Hamburgers And French Fries Are Available.

It has long been recognized that there exists a strong association between cognitive abilities and dietary consumption. Nevertheless, recent research indicates that the relationship between these variables might be considerably more significant and immediate than previously believed. Indeed, recent research indicates that a correlation may exist between the metabolism and various mood and cognitive impairment disorders. As an illustration, individuals who experience depression have a likelihood that exceeds 60% of developing type-2 diabetes. Individuals diagnosed with type-2 diabetes have a twofold increased risk of developing dementia. This implication suggests that the adage, 'You are what you eat,' possesses a depth and significance that may not be readily apparent. What is the cause of this phenomenon? Why do indulgent culinary items, characterized by their tempting flavors, delectable tastes, and irresistibly appetizing nature, exert such detrimental consequences on our well-being? (I am primarily referring to fast food, although not exclusively; it should be noted, however, that not all palatable food is inherently harmful.) The solution may be found in the extravagances.

Processed foods possess an exorbitant level of intricacy. It is my strong belief that had the resources allocated to the investigation of unhealthy food alternatives been redirected towards a more constructive endeavor such as the development of an optimal human diet, our collective physical fitness, well-being, and cognitive abilities would by now have reached exceptional levels. Regrettably, this is not the scenario. On the contrary, extensive research is conducted to determine the optimal degree of crispiness in potato chips or the most gratifying permutations of flavors. The aforementioned actions are undertaken with a singular objective in mind: to enhance the addictive properties of junk food.

There exist numerous rationales for our fondness towards unhealthy food options. It has been extensively devised to gratify certain fundamental aspirations within us, all the while leaving us yearning for further fulfillment. As an illustration, it is possible that you find yourself favoring the crisp texture of a certain brand of chips while harboringa distaste for another." Hence, solely on the basis of this fact, it is highly probable that you would opt to purchase the former and refrain from purchasing the latter, despite their equal taste. These seemingly inconsequential intricacies demand significant financial investments from companies, all aimed at determining what stimuli your mind perceives as gratifying and subsequently presenting it to you in an aesthetically pleasing manner.

Palatability constitutes an additional crucial element. The flavors of unhealthy and processed food are not derived from natural sources; rather, they are meticulously designed to deceive the human brain into perceiving them as exceptionally delightful. The majority of unhealthy foods exhibit a significantly saturated flavor profile that engenders a heightened sense of desire for additional consumption. Simultaneously, it is unlikely for one to grow fatigued with it due to its meticulous design that maintains an air of novelty and intrigue, regardless of its regular consumption. Consequently, it does not elicit the typical reaction associated with repetitious consumption.

Additionally, it should be noted that numerous types of unhealthy food items tend to "vanish" without a trace, providing you with the desired flavor while deceitfully convincing your brain that you have not consumed any calories, despite the fact that you actually have. These are merely a handful of illustrations, with countless additional instances in existence. Fast food items are indistinguishable; the hamburgers and fries that are frequently consumed for lunch adhere to the same standardized recipe, which accounts for their consistent appeal, irrespective of how frequently they are consumed. Nevertheless, the responsibility lies, in part, with our cognitive faculties for manifesting a gradual adaptability towards change.

The matter at hand is that during the Prehistoric era, there was a scarcity of readily accessible food items that were high in calories, fat, carbohydrates, and salt. Hence, we have cultivated a compulsion to seek out and derive pleasure from such experiences. The natural course of events conveys a message of approval, signifying one's commendable efforts. As previously mentioned, it was imperative for us to bear in mind the foods that promote our well-being and those that do not. The culinary items that were savored and provided us with delightful experiences were generally of exceptional quality. Nevertheless, in contemporary times, this is largely untrue. The identical regulation is upheld, albeit its culmination can primarily be ascribed to meticulously crafted flavors. In this manner, your mind continues to perceive commendable achievement despite the physical challenges your body encounters. The functioning of your brain is inclined towards an inherent drive to continuously seek additional sustenance, ensuring its acquisition and storage, primarily due to the prevalent scarcity of food throughout the greater part of human civilization. Given that nutrition is now easily accessible, the need to hunt or struggle for it has diminished considerably (unless one is employed as a hunter or fighter). However, this change inadvertently poses a challenge as the brain is not yet accustomed to this new reality. When this is compounded with the remarkable equilibrium that junk and fast food manufacturers achieve in terms of flavor, sensation, and contentment, it culminates in a profoundly detrimental way of living.

These foods give rise to numerous impacts that become apparent only upon discontinuation of their consumption. As an illustration, it is noteworthy that the consumption of a donut has the potential to rapidly elevate one's glucose levels to atypical levels. In such instances, the pancreas secretes insulin to determine the appropriate course of action regarding the glucose, either providing nourishment to the cells or directing the liver to store the surplus as glycogen in adipose tissue. Due to the excessive quantity of sugar, which is typically not immediately usable, it is stored. This proposition appears favorable, does it not? You obtain a substantial amount of energy, and it has been empirically demonstrated that insulin effectively enhances cognitive functions related to memory and learning. Therefore, this arrangement is mutually beneficial, correct? Well, yeah, not really. The issue lies in the rapid increase and subsequent decline of sugar and insulin levels, resulting in a deficiency that prompts you to seek another remedy. It entails a self-perpetuating cycle that can ultimately result in enduring harm such as insulin resistance or even the development of type-2 diabetes.

Hamburgers, French fries, and other high-fat fast food options are equally unfavorable. Research conducted in rodent models has demonstrated the potential to impair the hypothalamus, a pivotal brain region responsible for various functions such as mood and appetite regulation, as well as the previously mentioned hippocampus and other significant brain regions. Once more, these conclusions derive from scientific research conducted on rodents. Nevertheless, are you genuinely prepared to take such a gamble? These types of diets have been associated with diseases such as Alzheimer's and other forms of dementia typically ascribed to the elderly. It is highly possible that the food is the cause. It is hardly astonishing that substances can cause the blockage of arteries, elevate cholesterol levels, and contribute to a multitude of additional health hazards. Moreover, they inflict harm upon several organs, including the brain.

Would you be able to address this matter? Yes, yes you can. Cease your actions! It is not an overly arduous task. Typically, it requires approximately one week to completely overcome the habit (and by "overcome," I specifically refer to the addictive nature experienced by myself and numerous individuals). It is imperative that you cultivate practices that will facilitate the eradication of this detrimental lifestyle, and foster the adoption of a more wholesome and nourishing one. If not for the sake of your physical well-being and overall health, then prioritize it for the benefit of your mental cognition and memory. Ultimately, that is the defining factor in shaping your identity. Do not underestimate its value.

Eight: A Methodical Approach to Practicing Mindful Eating

This is devoted to presenting a systematic methodology for addressing binge eating, overeating, methods for cultivating self-discipline, techniques for practicing meditation, straightforward daily routines lasting just five minutes to incorporate mindful eating into your daily routine, and additional practices."

A multitude of captivating methodologies constitute the concept of mindful eating. Concretely, the process of practicing mindful eating commences with the act of grocery shopping. The food has already undergone multiple stages, starting from its initial production until its placement on the shelves of the grocery store. Nevertheless, it is imperative that you commence with conscientious food and grocery procurement.

1. Mastering the Art of Conscious Shopping

Learn to shop smartly. It is advisable to refrain from engaging in grocery shopping while experiencing hunger. The sensation of hunger can compel one to make less optimal food choices, particularly favoring fast foods, since the mind perceives them as an immediate means to appease cravings. Refrain from purchasing frozen goods. Remain within the sections dedicated to fresh food. Eliminate all the processed food present within your household. Presented herein are several prudent suggestions that shall assist you in carrying out your grocery shopping with a mindful approach:

Adhere to the periphery of the supermarket – The majority of supermarkets possess relatively comparable configurations. The arrangement of merchandise in most supermarkets and grocery stores typically follows a standardized format, encompassing diverse categories such as produce, fresh foods (including fruits, vegetables, dairy, and meat), baked goods, and processed foods.

The periphery of the supermarket is usually designated for perishable goods such as produce and fresh foods. The center of the market typically caters to processed foods, as their prolonged shelf life can be attributed to the incorporation of preservatives. Hence, by deliberately adhering to the boundary, opportunities to acquire processed foods are restricted, thereby increasing the likelihood of acquiring solely nutritious ingredients.

Opt for a handbasket as an alternative to a shopping cart – This method parallels the concept of selecting a smaller plate to consume meals mindfully, as previously mentioned in the dedicated to mindful eating versus. mindless eating. Upon encountering a partially occupied shopping cart that is functionally adequate, it is probable that your mind will experience a sense of discontent, compelling you to acquire more than necessary.

Conversely, upon observing a handbasket replete with items, one's cognitive and emotional state will be imbued with a sense of contentment derived from the shopping endeavor, thereby fostering a tendency to procure solely essential food items. Consider utilizing a handbasket when engaging in grocery shopping, as it represents an efficacious means of fostering mindfulness during the shopping process.

Familiarize yourself with the information displayed on food labels - Acquiring knowledge in effectively interpreting food labels can significantly contribute to making wise food choices. Please exercise caution and be aware of the structural makeup of the object you have selected. Please review the suggested serving size and calorie content of the product, taking note that occasionally the calorie count may be provided for a smaller serving than the recommended portion size, requiring additional calculations on your part. Additionally, take into consideration the incorporation of additives and preservatives, among other factors.

It is imperative that one exercises caution while purchasing sauces, masala mixes, and similar products. A significant portion of these items probably contain preservatives as well as elevated levels of sugar and salt in order to enhance their delectable flavor.

Once more, it is important to emphasize that engaging in mindful shopping does not imply that you should abstain from selecting the item of your choice. It is imperative to develop an awareness of one's purchasing choices. The key lies in the fact that when the human mind is aware of its actions, it tends to instinctively opt for the healthier alternative. Practicing conscientious shopping generally offers your mind an opportunity to carefully assess all factors before making a well-considered decision.

Adhere to purchasing genuine food items - Upon perusing the ingredients list, should you come across an unfamiliar or intricate ingredient name, it is prudent to refrain from making a purchase until conducting thorough research. Adhere to the nutritional choices that are beneficial for your well-being. The customary constituents encompass legumes, grains, proteins, fruits, and vegetables, among others. If preservation agents and artificial food colorings are present on the packaging, I recommend returning the product to its original location on the shelf.

2. Effortless Methods for Ceasing Episodes of Excessive Eating

Do not engage in the act of disregarding or intentionally avoiding the consumption of food during moments of hunger. By refraining from satisfying this natural bodily need, you initiate a neural response associated with stress within your cerebral cortex. Should you have the desire to consume a meal, it is prudent to exercise caution with respect to the corresponding emotion. Take a momentary pause to ascertain the presence of genuine hunger, and if you ascertain its authenticity, proceed to consume your meal with a mindful approach. Impositions serve as the principal catalyst for cravings. Therefore, it is prudent to refrain from imposing limitations, but rather to adopt a mindful approach.

Exercise kindness and compassion towards yourself - Often, following a bout of excessive eating, it is probable that you will experience feelings of shame regarding your actions. This mindset merely perpetuates a pattern of engaging in excessive eating episodes, as, in the absence of appropriate intervention, the individual resorts solely to food as a source of solace. Hence, to initiate the process, cease experiencing guilt. Rather, extend yourself compassion and kindness. In the event that your closest companion made an error, would you respond with severity towards them? Apply that identical conduct to oneself as well.

Adverse emotions and self-judgmental attitudes further impede your ability to comprehend the underlying factors contributing to your binge eating behavior. By adopting a practice of mindfulness, it is probable that you will discern the underlying cause of your difficulties.

Eliminate all indulgent food items from your kitchen and refrigerator – Although this measure may not entirely eradicate your binge eating tendencies, it can serve as a positive initial action. It facilitates the gradual and steady development of intuitive eating patterns, particularly concerning indulgent preferences.

For instance, if you experience a sense of insecurity regarding ice cream, ensure that your residence is devoid of any inventory of the aforementioned product. It exemplifies a commendable display of assistance and should not be perceived as a flaw. Recognizing the issue at hand is the initial stage towards conquering it.

Eliminating temptations allows individuals to attain greater mastery over their superfluous cravings. It would be imprudent to retain a substantial quantity of fry packages within your kitchen cupboard given your fondness for them and the need to overcome your inclination towards excessive eating. It is akin to granting an intruder access to your secure vault, even in the absence of immediate coercion or threat.

Please make sure your meal includes all the necessary nutrients. Once again, being mindful will prove beneficial in this regard. Prior to commencing your meal, it is advisable to inspect your plate and verify the presence of essential nutrients in your food. Ensure that you are consuming adequate amounts of carbohydrates, proteins, fats, vitamins, and minerals.

Frequently, the human body resorts to binge eating as a signal of inadequate nourishment. Presented here are a few illustrative instances:

• In the eventuality of bodily dehydration or insufficient Vitamin C levels, individuals may experience a penchant for confectionery items.

• A preference for high-sodium foods may suggest a deficiency in electrolytes such as potassium, sodium, zinc, or magnesium.

• In the event of suboptimal levels of Vitamin B12 or iron, individuals may experience a profound sense of depleted energy along with an inclination towards excessive eating.

Hence, it is crucial to ensure that you are receiving adequate quantities of all fundamental macronutrients and micronutrients required for optimal bodily function.

Avoid excessive engagement in high-intensity physical activities - It is frequently observed that individuals with compulsive eating issues engage in rigorous exercise routines as a means to alleviate their feelings of remorse. Additionally, a significant number of individuals have a tendency to escalate their levels of physical activity in an effort to prepare themselves for a session of indulgence without experiencing feelings of remorse.

This methodology can prove to be significantly counterproductive as indulgent overeating cannot be compensated for by engaging in exercise at a human-equivalent level. It is probable that you will experience increased anger and self-disappointment due to the inability to meet impractical expectations, thus perpetuating a cycle of overeating. I would recommend adhering to low-intensity physical activities such as walking, yoga, or stair climbing for optimal results.

Employ mindfulness techniques to cultivate awareness of your thoughts, emotions, and the inner wisdom conveyed by your heart and mind. Practicing conscientious eating is an excellent method for comprehending the signals your body emits, enabling you to accurately discern between genuine hunger and emotional hunger resulting from stress.

Take a moment to introspect whether you are experiencing hunger, anger, loneliness, or fatigue, employing the acronym "HALT." By understanding the underlying causes of your cravings, you will enhance your readiness to confront and resist episodes of binge eating, thus discovering effective strategies to combat them.

You're Body

Comprehending the mechanisms of one's own body is a highly intricate matter, thus it is prudent to simplify this by employing readily understandable language.

Your physique is truly a marvel of scientific inquiry, sparking significant deliberation around its mere existence. However, attaining a comprehensive comprehension of its functionality is not an insurmountable endeavor, provided one adopts a logical mindset when contemplating the underlying mechanisms.

For this particular segment of the book, I invite you to contemplate the notion of food as fuel, more specifically, the substance equivalent to the one utilized to power automobiles.

Think like this-

Petrol = Food

Let us further deconstruct this scenario: assuming you operate a gasoline-powered vehicle, when refueling, you wouldn't consider introducing diesel fuel, would you?

This is a common occurrence wherein individuals provide inadequate nourishment to their bodies on a daily basis. For instance, when one experiences hunger and only has the option of consuming leftover curry from the previous night or a chocolate bar, they proceed to hastily consume either of these options while anticipating optimal bodily function.

Have you ever pondered the reason behind your persistent fatigue, frequent skin blemishes, and potentially excessive perspiration? Have you had an epiphany or realization yet? Well it should of!

Many individuals I encounter attribute it to excessive stress and extended working hours; however, I perceive this justification to be inadequate.

Stress is a consequence of subjecting the body to enduring pressure and maintaining an unhealthy diet. Consequently, stress results in a deviation from our typical behavior, leading us to seek out high-fat foods for sustenance. Please trust me when I assert that you have inadvertently activated the self-destruct mechanism. Consuming these high-fat foods results in a gradual adaptation of our brains, leading to addiction to these cravings. Unfortunately, indulging in such foods not only interferes with our sleep patterns but also perpetuates a constant state of irritability.

It is an incessant cycle that we struggle to disrupt. I implore you to attempt an alternative approach when you experience the compulsion to indulge in a beverage or meal laden with excessive sugar and caffeine. Instead, turn on the cold tap and consume a large glass of refreshingly icy water. I am confident that you will experience an improved sense of well-being.

Initially, when I transitioned from consuming cola or energy drinks to water, I harbored doubts and questioned the efficacy of water in providing the necessary energy. I found it difficult to fathom how a seemingly inconsequential, transparent liquid sourced from taps could fulfill my energy requirements.

Fascinating information: the human body is composed of approximately 70% water. When one becomes dehydrated, the body naturally desires hydration, which is often satisfied by consuming beverages with high sugar and caffeine content. Due to the state of dehydration, fatigue results, and over an extended duration, this is the ideology that has been ingrained in our minds.

This situation is fundamentally incorrect and encompasses various levels of impropriety, individuals.

Indeed, while momentarily providing a surge of vigor, the subsequent decline in vitality becomes apparent within approximately an hour. It is imperative to acknowledge that water abounds with numerous essential nutrients, rendering its optimal consumption crucial. Water facilitates the elimination of toxins from your body. Insufficient water intake can result in the accumulation of substances that impede normal bodily functions. The kidneys, which function as the filtration system, depend on an adequate water supply to effectively flush out harmful toxins. Symptoms such as heartburn and restlessness often indicate a state of dehydration, where the body is lacking sufficient water.

In addition, it is worth noting that dehydration has the potential to result in a significant decrease in concentration, up to 40%. It is imperative to keep in mind that the quality of our performance and functioning greatly relies on the fuel we consume.

Before proceeding, allow me to emphasize the importance of water by reiterating its significance and benefits.

The diet we consume influences our physical appearance significantly. For instance, an individual who consistently consumes chocolate throughout their lifetime may appear emaciated due to a heightened metabolic rate. However, internally, their organs may be encased in adipose tissue, resulting in poor skin condition and potentially exhibiting extreme moodiness.

Similar to water, your body absorbs the nutrients from the food you consume. If you consume foods with high sugar content, your body attempts to eliminate the excessive nutrients, resulting in skin issues or digestive disturbances.

Nourishment is the driving force behind our productivity, therefore it is unwise to compromise your potential by consuming nutritionally inadequate items such as a oily kebab or pizza.

Allow me to offer an additional suggestion: The consumption of sugar can lead to the accumulation of fat in the body. While a small portion may be utilized as an energy source, the majority is transformed into adipose tissue. The extensive usage of artificially produced sugar is remarkably detrimental to health, making its lack of prohibition rather surprising.

There exists a prevalent fallacy within the realm of dietary practices, which holds that consuming fatty foods inevitably leads to the accumulation of body fat. It is of paramount importance to underscore the profound inaccuracy of this belief. There exist two distinct categories of fat: saturated fat and unsaturated fat.

Many experts consider saturated fat, commonly known as sat fat, to be significantly detrimental to one's health as it tends to adhere to the body and is notoriously challenging to eliminate. Dietary fat plays a crucial role in maintaining optimal health as it provides the essential building blocks for your digestive system, incorporating vital nutrients necessary for overall bodily function and stability.

Allow me to elaborate on this matter to the best of my abilities. I would like to request the complete elimination of calories. May I inquire about the rationale behind this decision? The reason for this is due to its lack of significance. I assure you of its insignificance.

The utilization of calorie-based guidelines by the government serves as a means of assuring individuals that adherence to recommended intake limits will yield satisfactory outcomes, regardless of their dietary choices. However, this approach is fundamentally flawed and entails systemic disadvantages.

In general, it holds true that a pizza with a higher fat content will contain more calories. It is worth noting that individuals often focus solely on the calorie count when evaluating their dietary choices. For instance, if someone were to consume a pizza that contributes to only 14% of their recommended daily calorie intake, they might mistakenly interpret this as permissible to consume six pizzas daily without consequence. Upon reflection, how could that have been considered logical?

It is the underlying cause of our burgeoning obesity crisis, as misguided information is being imparted to children. Parents imparting what they perceive as the appropriate skills to their children, albeit inaccurately. It represents an imminent threat that is poised to detonate, and the bubble is on the brink of collapse. My mother consistently emphasized the notion that one should not leave the dining table until their plate is completely empty. While I do not attribute my current physique solely to her influence, I must acknowledge that her approach significantly contributed to it. Hence, I urge individuals to consider reducing portion sizes. A young child will not consume equivalent quantities as an adult; as an individual partakes in greater amounts of food, their stomach expands and prompts the brain to send signals of increased hunger. Consequently, one may unintentionally undergo a significant increase in body size, despite adhering to dietary guidelines and fulfilling their body's demands.

Two: The Interconnected Relationship between the Heart and Brain

Eventually, we shall realize that the heart's righteousness will always be compromised if the intellect is entirely misguided. Man can attain his true potential only by uniting his intellect and morality - his capacity for thinking and his inherent goodness.

Dr. Martin Luther King, Jr.

From a health standpoint, it appears that the adage, "follow your head or follow your heart," may not be entirely true.

Contemporary studies are increasingly revealing significant connections between cardiovascular well-being and cognitive vitality, indicating that individuals who consume foods designed to promote heart health are often characterized by exceptional cognitive acuity and overall robust mental faculties.

In this section, we shall explore the correlation between the cardiovascular system and the central nervous system, elucidate the dietary choices that enhance cardiovascular well-being, and analyze the extensive array of advantages associated with adherence to heart-healthy nutritional plans.

Could you please elucidate the correlation between cardiovascular health and cognitive well-being?

Extensive evidence exhibits that an inadequate dietary pattern can contribute to the development of cardiovascular disease.[9] The accumulation of plaque in arteries, heightened workload on the heart, and elevated blood pressure are known repercussions of such a diet. All of these factors elevate the likelihood of experiencing cardiac events such as heart attacks, angina, and strokes, while also giving rise to the potential for your blood vessels to undergo blockages or develop diseases.

But how does this correlate with brain health?

The brain requires a substantial amount of oxygen. In the event that the supply ceases to be consistent, lasting longer than a few minutes without oxygen, the neurons within the brain will begin to experience cellular demise. On a continual basis, approximately one litre of blood traverses through the cerebral region of your body per minute, thereby facilitating the exchange of crucial gases and nutrients within the extensive network of around 400 miles of capillaries.

Blood supply is key. In the event of a stroke, there is a cessation of blood flow to a certain region of the brain, leading to ensuing damage or cessation of function, which may result in enduring cerebral impairment. This connection represents the most immediate and potentially distressing association between your cardiovascular system and the well-being of your brain.

Vascular dementia may arise as a consequence of an isolated stroke event, though it is not invariably the case. It may arise due to cerebral vasoconstriction or multiple transient ischaemic attacks (TIAs), resulting in transient reductions in cerebral blood flow. Both of these conditions are intricately connected to cardiovascular well-being.

Research conducted on individuals diagnosed with Alzheimer's disease has revealed that their cerebral blood flow is frequently diminished to a considerable extent, accompanied by notable vascular impairment. In precise terms, researchers are postulating that adequate cerebral blood flow plays a vital role in the elimination of tubular proteins, thereby preventing the accumulation of 'neurofibrillary tangles' within the brain. These tangled, tubular structures comprised of tau proteins commonly manifest in the neurons of individuals affected by Alzheimer's disease.

Heart issues and brain issues share common risk factors. Furthermore, the presence of these risk factors in younger individuals poses detrimental effects on their brain health in later stages of life.

Obesity is linked to accelerated cerebral atrophy. It has been observed that there is a decline in mass that commences during middle age, and this can notably impact the region linked to memory if an individual is obese.

Elevated blood pressure poses a clear risk factor for stroke, particularly haemorrhagic stroke where blood vessels that have been weakened rupture and result in bleeding within the brain. However, even in the absence of such an event, hypertension escalates the likelihood of developing dementia in later stages of life.

Although high cholesterol is not considered a risk factor for vascular dementia, it does pose a risk for the onset of Alzheimer's disease later in life if one's cholesterol levels are elevated during mid-life.

Diabetes, in both its types, can induce alterations in blood vessels that impede blood circulation to the brain. Consequently, this can impede cognitive abilities during middle age and escalate the likelihood of developing Alzheimer's disease and vascular dementia.

Dementia and cognitive impairment are often erroneously perceived as issues that primarily concern individuals in advanced age, leading to the assumption that they do not impact younger individuals. It is plausible that one may not perceive its consequences during adolescence, however, it is during this pivotal phase that one initiates the establishment of a foundation for the trajectory of their cognitive well-being. One begins to cultivate problems when they possess a sense of invulnerability and lack awareness of potential challenges.

The ongoing progression of what transpires within your future cognitive functions has been evident for a considerable duration.

A comprehensive investigation, published in the year 2021,[10], analyzed data from a sample consisting of 15,001 individuals aged 18–95, encompassing a wide spectrum of age groups. Given the extensive range of data collected, this study can be regarded as a substantial cohort. In the realm of scientific investigations, substantial evidence is inherently more persuasive when derived from extensive sample sizes. Should the populations under scrutiny be insufficient in magnitude, the margin of error may drastically escalate, ultimately rendering the outcomes statistically irrelevant.

The research examined various factors including cardiovascular health, body mass index, fasting glucose, total cholesterol, as well as assessing global cognition and processing speed. They employed a selection of rigorous assessments, namely the Modified Mini-Mental State Examination (3MS), which assesses verbal capacities such as attention, memory, and language, and the Digit Symbol

Substitution Test (DSST), a paper-and-pencil test that measures motor speed and visuoperceptual functions. The study also took into account demographic variables, educational attainment, and cohort effects.

The study's results were of grave nature, as it highlighted a notable correlation between cardiovascular risk factors throughout an individual's lifespan, particularly during early adulthood, and a heightened susceptibility to cognitive decline in later stages of life. This finding merits particular attention.

This is a matter of utmost significance that warrants careful consideration as it pertains to every individual. In the phase of early adulthood, there continues to be ongoing brain development, as evidenced by studies examining chess proficiency. It has been observed that the capacity for brain processing power tends to augment until around the age of 45 for certain individuals. Thus, even amidst the periods wherein you perceive enhancements in your cognitive abilities or the pinnacle of your brain's performance, the absence of a healthy heart would inevitably undermine the well-being of your brain.

The unbroken and crucial connection between the heart and the brain extends beyond the mere prevention of debilitating disorders such as dementia. Consistently upholding and enhancing the overall well-being of the cardiovascular system, which serves as the intermediary for supplying blood to the brain, is the key to expediting cognitive processes, enhancing memory, and achieving superior cognitive performance.

An Understanding Of The End Date

Welcome to your journey with the MIND diet! Whether you are familiar with the MIND diet and seeking to expand your knowledge or are newly introduced to it, this will provide you with a comprehensive understanding of the fundamental aspects of this dietary approach.

In this chapter, I will provide an elucidation of the research underpinning the MIIND diet, facilitate your comprehension of the correlation between dietary choices and cognitive wellbeing, and furnish you with guidance on the selection of foods to incorporate into your regular regimen, as well as those that warrant restriction.

What is the definition of the MIND Diet?

Martha Clare Morris, ScD, and her research team from Rush University Medical Center in Chicago have devised a dietary pattern based on previous studies investigating the impact of diet on brain health, as initially documented in September 2015 in the journal Alzheimer's & Dementia. Referred to as the Mediterranean-DASH Diet Intervention for Neurodegenerative Delay (MIND), this groundbreaking study revealed that individuals who achieved the highest scores on the MIND diet demonstrated a significantly slower deterioration in cognitive function over a span of 4.7 years, as compared to those who obtained the lowest scores on the MIND diet. In the same year, Morris and her team published a subsequent study which demonstrated that strict adherence to the MIND diet was linked to a notable reduction of 52 percent in the risk of developing Alzheimer's disease over a period of 4.5 years.

MIND represents the acronym for Mediterranean-DASH InterventionforNeurodegenerativeDelay.

As evident from its name, the diet is a fusion of two widely recognized dietary patterns - the Mediterranean diet and the DASH diet. The Mediterranean diet is derived from the culinary customs observed in Mediterranean nations. It underscores the importance of incorporating nutritious fats like extra-virgin olive oil and nuts, as well as fresh fruits and vegetables, whole grains, and legumes into one's diet while restricting the intake of red meat and added sugars. Similar to the Mediterranean diet, the DASH (Dietary Approaches to Stop Hypertension) diet places emphasis on the consumption of fruits, vegetables, whole grains, and lean meats. Becauseitwasdevelopedtotreathypertension, italsolimitsdailysodiumintake.

Both the Mediterranean and DASH diets have been associated with improved brain health, hence it is unsurprising that the MIND diet incorporates many of their principles. What sets the MИИD diet apart is its emphasis on the specific foods and nutrients that have been proven to enhance and safeguard brain health while decreasing the likelihood of developing Alzheimer's disease and dementia.

For instance, while the Mediterranean diet includes a general recommendation to increase fruit consumption, the MIND diet specifically advises incorporating berries into one's diet multiple times per week due to research findings that indicate a correlation between berry consumption and improved cognitive function.

While further research is still being conducted on the MIND diet, additional studies have already demonstrated encouraging findings. For instance, an investigation conducted in 2019 among a sample of 1,220 adults revealed a pronounced correlation between increased adherence to the MIND diet and a decreased likelihood of experiencing cognitive impairment over a span of 12 years. A different study discovered a substantially diminished likelihood of developing or experiencing a slower advancement of Parkinson's disease over a period of 4.6 years.

As a registered dietitian and nutritionist with a strong interest in food and a background in research, I am of the opinion that not only does the MIND diet have advantages for brain health, but it can also serve as a highly fulfilling and nutritionally balanced approach to eating. My objective entails furnishing you with the necessary information and recipes to adhere to the MIND diet.

Gaining Insight into Alzheimer's, Dementia, and Cognitive Decline

In order to delve into the numerous advantages that the MIND diet may offer for enhancing brain health, it is crucial to obtain a comprehensive comprehension of the contrasting characteristics separating Alzheimer'sdisease, dementia, and cognitivedecline.

ALZHEIMER'S DISEASE

Alzheimer's disease is a degenerative neurological condition that is irreversible in nature. According to the National Institute on Aging, it is estimated that this condition impacts over five million individuals in the United States. One of the primary characteristics of Alzheimer's disease is the accumulation of atypical protein deposits that form plaques and tangles within the cerebral structure. Additionally, there is a lack of connectivity between nerve cells and, in more severe instances, even a reduction in brain volume. Symptoms encompass memory impairment, cognitive decline, disorientation, alterations in behavior, speech difficulties, lethargy, and progressively developing swallowing challenges. Due to the progressive nature of Alzheimer's disease, these symptoms tend to exacerbate and become increasingly apparent over time.

At present, researchers are uncertain regarding the etiology of Alzheimer's disease in the majority of individuals. Nevertheless, it is believed that it is probable a culmination of factors, encompassing genetics, environment, and lifestyle factors, which notably include nutrition. While a cure for Alzheimer's disease remains elusive, continuous research endeavors are being undertaken to explore potential treatment modalities and preventive measures.

DEMENTIA

Contrary to Alzheimer's, dementia is not a specific ailment but rather a cluster of symptoms indicative of a deterioration in cognitive function, such as memory loss or impaired concentration. Dementia can be conceptualized as a comprehensive framework encompassing multiple disorders that give rise to persistent memory impairment, including Alzheimer's disease. Infact, Alzheimer'sisthemostcommonformofdementia, accountingfor 50 to 70 percentofdementiacases.

The second most prevalent form of dementia is vascular dementia, which arises due to insufficient cerebral blood circulation. It may progress gradually over time or abruptly, such as in the aftermath of a stroke. Additional forms of dementia include Lewy body dementia, Parkinson's disease, Creutzfeldt-Jakob disease, Wernicke-Korsakoff syndrome, and Huntington's disease. Additionally, illnesses such as HIV and multiple sclerosis have the potential to induce dementia, particularly during advanced stages.

Although certain forms of cognitive decline, such as dementia caused by alcohol or drug abuse, may be reversible if promptly addressed, the vast majority of other types including vascular dementia, Alzheimer's disease, and Huntington's disease, lead to an irreversible deterioration of cognitive abilities.

COGNITIVE DECLINE

Cognitive decline refers to the general decrease in fundamental cognitive abilities. As one progresses in age, one may observe subtle alterations in their cognitive abilities, including intelligence, memory, concentration, verbal expression, reasoning, and/or processing speed. For instance, you might encounter challenges in recollecting the name of a location you previously visited. Despite being frustrating, individuals experiencing normal cognitive decline do not lose information; rather, it may simply take longer for their brain to retrieve it.

The positive aspect is that there exist methods not only for mitigating cognitive decline in older adults, but also for enhancing these cognitive processes. Promoting stress reduction, scheduling regular medical check-ups, engaging in activities that stimulate cognitive function, maintaining physical activity, and adhering to a diet abundant in antioxidants and healthy fats will all contribute to maintaining optimal brain health.

AssessingtheRiskFactors

Aside from the aging process, which is widely regarded as the most significant risk factor for cognitive decline and dementia, here are four of the foremost risk factors.

Familyhistory. Individuals with a familial predisposition to Alzheimer's disease are at an elevated risk of developing the condition. While it is not possible to alter one's genetic makeup, individuals are able to lower their risk by implementing lifestyle modifications and effectively managing other health conditions.

Heartdisease. Heart disease, along with elevated blood pressure and high levels of cholesterol, impairs blood circulation to the brain, resulting in neuronal damage, impaired brain function, and cognitive decline. Fortunately, one can enhance cardiovascular health via the consistent engagement in physical exercise, consumption of a well-rounded diet, maintenance of a healthy body weight, and abstention from smoking.

Headinjury. Recent research has revealed that traumatic brain injury is a significant risk factor associated with Alzheimer's disease and dementia. This connection can be attributed to the fact that brain injuries have the potential to cause irreversible damage or death of brain cells. Although it may be impossible to completely prevent accidents, you can decrease the overall likelihood or severity of a brain injury by wearing a helmet during sports activities, fastening your seatbelt, and implementing safety measures in your home to minimize the risk of falls.

Tobacco usage and excessive alcohol consumption. Both have been associated with an elevated susceptibility to cognitive decline and dementia. To mitigate your risk, abstain completely from smoking and consume alcohol in moderation.

1 – Evaluating Personal Consciousness

Your sense of observation

There may be individuals within your midst who engage in dishonest practices, however, it is crucial to bear in mind that resorting to cheating will impede your comprehension of the true essence of mindfulness and prolong the learning process. I engaged in dishonest conduct, yet I progressed beyond that because the sole individual I deceived was none other than myself. Please locate a seating area with which you are not acquainted. This location has the potential to be situated within a park. It is possible to be situated within a workplace setting, however, optimal outcomes are consistently achieved by fostering proximity to the natural environment. Please briefly observe your surroundings before gently closing your eyes.

May I inquire about the observations you made upon surveying your surroundings? Please provide a detailed depiction of the visual experience stored within your mental consciousness. Did the sky have cloud cover? Were any flowers present, and if so, what was their color? Did a particular color dominate? Did you observe any notably exquisite elements in your vicinity? Were there any people? Please provide a thorough and detailed description using your imagination.

In a televised program, individuals were presented with a sequential arrangement of items being conveyed along a belt. They were granted permission to retain those items provided they could commit them to memory; nevertheless, there were numerous instances of oversight. In your particular situation, it is imperative that you provide a comprehensive account of your observations prior to unveiling the truth by opening your eyes. It is a common tendency for individuals to overlook or fail to notice certain things. There might have been conspicuous elements that should have been incorporated into your conceptualization of that location, but that you overlooked. Such a circumstance arises due to the absence of prior conditioning to enable your mind to exist in the present moment, fully conscious of its surroundings.

This publication will elucidate the process through which this achievement is attained, as the acquisition of maximal advantages from one's encounters necessitates the cultivation of a state of mindful composure. It may require a brief adjustment period, but the endeavor will prove to be worthwhile in due course.

Observing people around you

Engaging in the practice of observing individuals in your vicinity can facilitate a broader understanding of circumstances. Observe the manner in which individuals exuding joy effortlessly draw companionship, whereas despondency often repels them. Individuals who acquire knowledge through the act of observing others possess the ability to consciously determine their desired presentation within any given temporal context. They gain consciousness of their deficiencies and strive to maximize their personal growth and development in all circumstances.

What does that mean?

This implies that your state of happiness is crucial for maintaining good physical and emotional well-being, both for yourself and those in your proximity. In the event that one experiences discomfort with regards to their current circumstances or personal state, it is likely that they will exhibit a diminished level of engagement in the present moment. Observe the manner in which individuals engage with one another. Consider the activities you would be inclined to abstain from. Through careful observation, it is possible to discern the errors individuals make, and it is conceivable that you might possess some of these shortcomings as well.

The sense of self-assurance that one acquires through the practice of mindfulness is truly remarkable. Look at confident people. The demeanor exhibited by individuals with less confidence contrasts with that displayed by them. Note their body language. It is not a matter of their external appearance in terms of aesthetic attractiveness, but rather their internal disposition. Certain individuals exhibit a greater propensity for mindfulness and a heightened awareness of their interpersonal interactions. These individuals exude a sense of genuine joy and satisfaction, possessing the ability to effortlessly captivate a room's attention. Their appeal lies in the serenity of their comportment and the unadulterated joy they exude, a manifestation of genuine and unrestrained emotions.

Significant insights can be acquired through the act of observation. In the forthcoming chapters, we shall guide you through mindfulness exercises, aiming to facilitate your ability to fully embrace the present moment and optimize its quality, thus leading to an unparalleled experience. Mindfulness entails recognizing that the present moment is finite, and by acknowledging this truth, one can imbue the present with a sense of fulfillment, since neglecting to do so would render the moment irretrievable and forfeit its potential.

Primarily, mindfulness entails maintaining a keen sense of self-awareness throughout all your actions. However, engaging in these observation exercises will aid in identifying the aspects within yourself that demand recognition, thereby facilitating personal growth. Mindfulness is not judgmental. It encompasses the act of observing and accepting oneself with simplicity. Once one embarks on this practice, they will discover that life's multitude of blessings will manifest before them, leading to profound happiness and contentment.

A study conducted on the MIND Diet

Numerous research studies have been conducted to investigate the potential effects of the MIND diet in terms of Alzheimer's disease prevention and other forms of dementia.

The correlation between the MIND Diet and a decelerated rate of cognitive decline was observed in a study conducted on a cohort of 960 elderly individuals enrolled in the Rush Memory and Aging Project. The participants adhered to the MIND diet over a duration of nearly five years, with their cognitive functionality being assessed on an annual basis throughout the study.

Scientists have discovered that maintaining a strong fidelity to the MIND diet is associated with a deceleration of cognitive deterioration commonly observed in the aging process. In reality, they concluded that the outcomes were comparable to an individual attaining the cognitive abilities of a person who was 7 1/2 years younger. The participants demonstrated notable improvements in both their overall cognitive scores and their individual subsection scores. The various components encompassed within this category consist of episodic memory, semantic memory, and perceptual speed.

The MIND Diet was found to be associated with a decreased incidence of Alzheimer's disease: Furthermore, another study was conducted by the same researchers responsible for the aforementioned study. Their objective was to ascertain whether the MIND diet not only mitigated the pace of cognitive deterioration but also yielded reduced incidences of Alzheimer's disease.

In this study, the researchers specifically examined three distinct dietary patterns, namely the MIND diet, the Mediterranean diet, and the DASH diet. They assessed the degree of adherence to those diets (that is, the strictness with which the diets were followed) and subsequently identified the individuals who later developed Alzheimer's disease.

The researchers also took into account other characteristics of the participants that have previously been associated with the risk of dementia, such as their levels of physical activity, age, gender, educational attainment, obesity, low BMI, and medical history including high blood pressure, stroke, or diabetes. This measure was implemented in order to mitigate the likelihood that factors aside from diet were significantly influencing the outcomes of the research.

The findings of the study indicated that individuals who adhered closely to the MIND diet experienced a 53 percent reduction in the likelihood of developing Alzheimer's disease, as compared to those who did not adhere to the diet. The MIND diet boasts a particularly positive aspect, namely that even partial adherence to its guidelines (termed as 'moderate adherence' by the study's authors) was still associated with a notable 35 percent decrease in the risk of developing Alzheimer's disease.

Curiously, there was a reduction in the risk of dementia when individuals adhered closely to both the DASH diet and the Mediterranean diet. However, it should be noted that only a moderate level of compliance with these two diets did not significantly decrease the occurrence of Alzheimer's disease.

The 2017 Alzheimer's Association International Conference featured presentations on the MIND diet, as well as other dietary patterns that have been correlated with enhanced cognitive function.

In a particular study, a nearly 30 to 35 percent decrease in the likelihood of experiencing cognitive impairment was observed in a cohort of approximately 6,000 elderly individuals who rigorously adhered to both the Mediterranean diet and the MIND diet. Adhering to either the MIND or the Mediterranean diet in a moderate manner was linked to a decrease of 18 percent in the likelihood of experiencing cognitive impairment.

An alternative formulation in formal tone could be: "The U.S.-based Women's Health Initiative Memory Study encompassed a sample size of over 7,000 women, with an average age of 71 years." Their adherence to the MIND diet was evaluated and subsequently classified as highly adherent (4th quartile) to minimally adherent (1st quartile). In contrast to the first quartile, the remaining three quartiles demonstrated a noteworthy decrease in the likelihood of developing dementia. Once more, the aforementioned observation solidifies the notion that achieving impeccable adherence to a nutritious dietary regimen might not be imperative in order to reap advantageous effects on our cognitive capacities.

Another research paper presented at the conference revealed a significant association between an inadequate dietary pattern and reduced brain volume. The size of the brain has previously been linked to the wellbeing and cognitive performance of the brain. In the case of Alzheimer's disease, there is a substantial reduction in brain volume. The primary focus of this study did not revolve specifically around the MIND diet, but instead emphasized the significance of maintaining a nutritious diet in general for the promotion of brain health.

GreekYogurt Breakfast Bowl

Ingredients

- 1 tsp honey
- 1 tbsp chopped nuts
- 1 cup Greek Yogurtplain
- 1/3 cup fresh fruit (or frozenfruitthat'sbeenthawed)

Instructions

1. Place the greekyogurtin a bowl, top withfruit, nuts and drizzle honey over the top

A Selection Of Food Items To Incorporate Into The Mind Diet

Behold, the MIND diet advocates for the following nourishments:

• Consume a minimum of six servings per week of green, leafy vegetables. This encompasses kale, spinach, cooked greens, as well as various salad options.

• All other vegetables: It is recommended to incorporate an additional vegetable into your daily diet along with the green leafy vegetables. Opt for non-starchy vegetables as they exhibit a high nutritional value while containing a minimal calorific content.

• Consumption of berries is recommended to occur at a minimum frequency of twice a week. While the published research solely focuses on strawberries, it is advisable to incorporate other berry varieties, such as blueberries, raspberries, and blackberries, into your diet to reap their antioxidant benefits.

- Nuts: Aim to consume at least five servings of nuts per week. The developers of the MIND diet do not specify the specific types of nuts to consume, but it is advisable to diversify the selection of nuts in order to obtain a range of nutrients.

- Utilize olive oil as the primary cooking oil.

- Incorporate a minimum of three servings of whole grains into your daily diet. Select whole grains such as oats, quinoa, brown rice, whole wheat pasta, and bread made entirely from whole wheat.

- Consume fish at a frequency of no less than once a week. It is advisable to opt for fatty fish varieties such as salmon, sardines, trout, tuna, and mackerel due to their abundant content of omega-3 fatty acids.

- Incorporate beans into a minimum of four meals per week. This encompasses all types of legumes, such as beans, lentils, and soybeans.

- Poultry: It is advised to consume chicken or turkey a minimum of two times per week. Please be advised that the consumption of fried chicken is not recommended according to the MIND diet guidelines.

- Wine consumption should be limited to no more than a single glass per day. Both red and white wine offer potential cognitive benefits to the brain. Nevertheless, extensive research has been centered on the compound resveratrol found in red wine, which shows potential in providing protection against Alzheimer's disease.

If you are unable to consume the desired quantity of servings, it is advised not to entirely discontinue the MIND diet. Extensive research has demonstrated that adhering to the MIND diet, even in moderation, is connected to a decreased likelihood of developing Alzheimer's disease. When adhering to the prescribed dietary regimen, you are not limited to the consumption of solely these 10 food items.

Nevertheless, adhering to the diet consistently may yield more favorable outcomes. Based on the findings of the research, it has been observed that increasing consumption of the 10 recommended foods while reducing intake of the foods to avoid is linked to a decreased likelihood of developing Alzheimer's disease, as well as an improvement in cognitive function over an extended period.

Food Items to Be Excluded on the MIND Diet

The MIND diet advocates for restrictions on the consumption of the following five foods:

• Limit consumption of butter and margarine to less than 1 tablespoon (approximately 14 grams) per day. Instead, consider employing olive oil as your primary culinary fat, and indulging by dipping your bread in fragrant olive oil infused with herbs.

- Cheese: It is advised by the MIND diet to restrict the consumption of cheese to a frequency of less than once per week.

- Red meat consumption should not exceed three servings per week. This encompasses all forms of beef, pork, lamb, and any derivatives derived from these types of meat.

- Fried food: The MIND diet strongly advises against the consumption of fried food, particularly the type commonly found in fast-food establishments. Please restrict your consumption to a frequency of less than once per week.

- Pastries and confections: This encompasses a majority of the processed unhealthy food options and desserts available. Ice cream, cookies, brownies, snack cakes, donuts, candies, and various other confections. Please endeavor to restrict these occurrences to a maximum of four instances per week.

Experts advocate for modulating the intake of these food items due to their high content of both saturated and trans fats. Research has established a strong correlation between trans fats and various health conditions, including cardiovascular disorders and even Alzheimer's disease. Nonetheless, the impact of saturated fat on health remains a subject of extensive debate within the field of nutrition. While the research regarding the relationship between saturated fats and heart disease lacks a definitive conclusion and remains a highly debated topic, studies conducted on animals as well as observations made on human subjects do indicate that excessive consumption of saturated fats is linked to compromised brain health.

A Weekly Exemplary Dietary Plan

Preparing meals for the MIND diet need not be overly complex. Presented below is a comprehensive seven-day meal plan to initiate your dietary journey:

Monday

- Morning meal: A serving of Greek yogurt accompanied by raspberries, garnished with a generous sprinkle of sliced almonds.

• Midday Meal: A Mediterranean salad composed of mixed greens and vegetables, accompanied by grilled chicken and served with a whole-wheat pita.

Formal alternative: • Evening meal: Burrito bowl consisting of brown rice, black beans, sautéed fajita vegetables, grilled chicken, salsa, and guacamole.

Tuesday

• Morning meal: Slices of whole wheat bread spread with almond butter, accompanied by savory scrambled eggs.

• Midday Meal: Sandwich made with grilled chicken, accompanied by blackberries and carrots.

Dinner will consist of a grilled salmon accompanied by a side salad dressed with olive oil and brown rice.

Wednesday

- Breakfast: A nutritious meal consisting of steel-cut oats topped with fresh strawberries, accompanied by hard-boiled eggs.

- Midday meal: A salad in the Mexican culinary style, composed of a combination of various lettuces, black beans, red onions, corn, grilled chicken, and a dressing made predominantly from olive oil.

- Dinner: A stir-fry dish made with chicken and a variety of vegetables served over a bed of brown rice.

Thursday

- Morning meal: Consuming Greek yogurt accompanied by peanut butter and banana.

- Lunch: oven-roasted trout served with sautéed collard greens and seasoned black-eyed peas.

Dinner: A dish consisting of whole-wheat spaghetti accompanied by turkey meatballs and marinara sauce, served with a side salad dressed with olive oil.

Friday

• Breakfast: A combination of wheat toast topped with avocado, alongside an omelet infused with the flavors of peppers and onions.

• Lunch: Chili prepared using ground turkey.

• Evening meal: Baked chicken seasoned with Greek herbs and spices, oven-roasted potatoes, accompanying side salad, whole wheat dinner roll.

Saturday

• Morning meal: Prepared oats soaked overnight accompanied by fresh strawberries.

Lunch will consist of fish tacos served on whole wheat tortillas, accompanied by brown rice and pinto beans.

- Evening meal: Grilled chicken gyro served on a whole-wheat pita, accompanied by a salad of fresh cucumber and tomato.

Sunday

- Breakfast option: Spinach frittata accompanied by sliced apple and peanut butter.

- Midday meal: A sandwich composed of tuna salad, served on whole wheat bread, accompanied by carrots and celery alongside a side of hummus.

- Evening meal: Chicken curry served with brown rice and lentils.

To adhere to the dietary guidelines of the MIND diet, it is permissible to consume a serving of wine alongside each evening meal. Nuts can also serve as an excellent choice for a snack. The majority of salad dressings available in retail outlets are not predominantly composed of olive oil; however, it is possible to effortlessly prepare your own salad dressing in the comfort of your own home. To prepare a basic balsamic vinaigrette, blend together three portions of extra virgin olive oil with one portion of balsamic vinegar. Incorporate a small amount of Dijon mustard, along with the requisite amount of salt and pepper, and proceed to thoroughly blend the ingredients.

The MIND Diet may have potential benefits in reducing oxidative stress and inflammation.

The existing research on the MIND diet has not been successful in elucidating its precise mechanisms. Nevertheless, the scientists responsible for formulating the dietary regimen posit that its potential efficacy could be attributed to its ability to mitigate oxidative stress and inflammation. Oxidative stress arises as a result of the accumulation of unstable molecules known as free radicals in significant quantities within the body. This frequently results in cellular damage. The brain is particularly susceptible to this type of injury. Inflammation is an innate bodily response triggered by injury and infection. However, when not appropriately regulated, inflammation can also exert detrimental effects and contribute to numerous chronic ailments. In conjunction, the combination of oxidative stress and inflammation can have significant adverse effects on the brain. In recent times, these have garnered attention in various interventions aimed at the prevention and treatment of Alzheimer's disease. Adhering to the Mediterranean and DASH dietary patterns is linked to reduced levels of oxidative stress and inflammation. As the MIND diet is a combination of these two dietary approaches, it is likely that the foods comprising the MIND diet also possess antioxidative and anti-inflammatory properties. The antioxidants present in berries, together with the vitamin E found in olive oil, green leafy vegetables, and nuts, are believed to confer positive effects on cognitive function by safeguarding the brain against oxidative stress. Furthermore, it should be noted that the omega-3 fatty acids present in fatty fish are widely recognized for their capacity to reduce inflammation within the brain, thereby potentially slowing down the rate of cognitive decline.

The Mind Diet has the potential to mitigate the presence of detrimental beta-amyloid proteins.

In addition, scientists posit that the MIND diet could potentially yield favorable effects on cognitive function by mitigating the levels of beta-amyloid proteins, which are known to be detrimental to the brain. Beta-amyloid proteins are naturally occurring protein fragments in the human body. Nonetheless, these substances have the potential to amass and generate plaques within the brain, thereby impeding the communication among brain cells and ultimately resulting in neural cell degeneration. Indeed, it is widely held among scientists that these plaques are a foremost factor contributing to the onset of Alzheimer's disease. Animal and laboratory experiments indicate that the antioxidants and vitamins present in numerous foods comprising the MIND diet possess the potential to inhibit the development of beta-amyloid plaques within the brain. In addition, the MIND diet also restricts the consumption of foods containing saturated and trans fats, as scientific research has indicated that these fats can lead to elevated levels of beta-amyloid protein in the brains of mice. Evidence from observational studies involving human subjects has revealed a significant correlation between the consumption of these fats and a twofold increase in the likelihood of developing Alzheimer's disease. Nevertheless, it is crucial to acknowledge that this form of investigation lacks the capacity to establish causal relationships. Additional research of a more rigorous nature is imperative in order to ascertain the precise ways in which the MIND diet could potentially enhance cognitive well-being.

www.ingramcontent.com/pod-product-compliance
Lightning Source LLC
Chambersburg PA
CBHW070030040426
42333CB00040B/1418